Soumia Benbernou
Nabil Ghomari
Rabah Kouadria

Diagnosis and management of cerebral venous thrombosis

Soumia Benbernou
Nabil Ghomari
Rabah Kouadria

Diagnosis and management of cerebral venous thrombosis

Cerebral venous thrombosis

ScienciaScripts

Imprint

Any brand names and product names mentioned in this book are subject to trademark, brand or patent protection and are trademarks or registered trademarks of their respective holders. The use of brand names, product names, common names, trade names, product descriptions etc. even without a particular marking in this work is in no way to be construed to mean that such names may be regarded as unrestricted in respect of trademark and brand protection legislation and could thus be used by anyone.

Cover image: www.ingimage.com

This book is a translation from the original published under ISBN 978-620-6-70250-4.

Publisher:
Sciencia Scripts
is a trademark of
Dodo Books Indian Ocean Ltd. and OmniScriptum S.R.L publishing group

120 High Road, East Finchley, London, N2 9ED, United Kingdom
Str. Armeneasca 28/1, office 1, Chisinau MD-2012, Republic of Moldova, Europe
Printed at: see last page
ISBN: 978-620-7-85117-1

Contents :

Abbreviations 2

1   INTRODUCTION 3

2   History and epidemiology : 4

3   DEFINITION : 5

4   ANATOMY : 5

5   PHYSIOLOGY AND PHYSIOPATOLOGY : 13

6   CLINICAL ASPECTS 15

7   RADIOLOGICAL DIAGNOSIS 18

8   Other examinations : 32

9   TOPOGRAPHICAL DIAGNOSIS 34

10   ETIOLOGIES AND RISK FACTORS FOR CTV 35

11   DIFFERENTIAL DIAGNOSIS OF TVC 44

12   THERAPEUTIC CARE : 45

13   MALIGNANT VENOUS THROMBOSIS 49

14 EVOLUTION AND PROGNOSIS : 49

14   CONCLUSION 51

BIBLIOGRAPHICAL REFERENCES 53

Appendices 56

Abbreviations

CVT: cerebral venous thrombosis

TPC: thrombophlebitis cerberus

CO: oral contraception

F: female

H: male

MH: meningeal hemorrhage

OC: cerebral edema

SC: cavernous sinus

SLD: right lateral sinus

LHS: left lateral sinus

LS: superior longitudinal sinus

SSgD: right sigmoid sinus

ST: transverse sinus

CT: computed tomography of the brain

MRA: magnetic resonance angiography

MRI: magnetic resonance imaging

VB: basilar vein.

VCI: internal cerebral vein.

HTIC: intracranial hypertension.

CSF: cerebrospinal fluid.

CRP: c reactin protein.

SA: week of amenorrhea.

1 INTRODUCTION

Cerebral venous thrombosis (CVT) or cerebral thrombophlebitis is an extremely rare cause of vascular headache. In recent years, they have been diagnosed with increasing frequency, thanks to the huge advances in medical imaging. The clinical spectrum and chronological course of the disease are varied. In its early stages, cerebral venous thrombosis often manifests as isolated headaches. Other clinical manifestations of cerebral venous thrombosis depend on the size and location of the thrombosed veins: epileptic seizures, focal deficits associated with bleeding due to venous congestion or infarction, signs of intracranial hypertension and psychic disorders. Thrombosis of the cavernous sinus occupies a special place, and may be accompanied by exophthalmos, conjunctival chemosis, oculomotor paralysis and sensory disturbances in the territory innervated by the first branch of the trigeminal nerve. From an etiological point of view, local causes, hereditary coagulation disorders, contraceptive use, pregnancy and the post-partum period are prominent in young patients. In elderly patients, DVT is often associated with tumors. Thanks to early diagnosis and timely treatment, the vast majority of patients are able to avoid sequelae.

2 History and epidemiology:

Cerebral venous thrombosis was first described by Ribes in 1825 [1]. For many years, CVT was considered an infectious disease, leading to occlusion of the superior sagittal sinus or superior longitudinal sinus, bilateral focal deficits, seizures, coma and finally death. It was the revolution in imaging procedures that made the reliable diagnosis of CVT possible in the first place, and contributed greatly to our understanding of the clinical picture.

In 1972, the first x-ray scanner was invented by British engineer God Frey new bold Hounsfield. Designed solely for cross-sectional imaging of the head, in particular the brain, without puncturing or opening the head, it gives us images of the cerebral ventricles and fluid spaces.

Cerebral CT scans can be used to recognize both normal and lesional aspects, whether traumatic (hematomas), vascular (strokes), tumoral, infectious, malformative or other.

Magnetic resonance imaging was developed in 1973, and quickly became the method of choice in many medical fields, particularly those related to the brain, thanks to the work of two inventors, Paul lanterbur and Peter Mansfield, who won the 2003 Nobel Prize for Physiology in Medicine.

The actual incidence of CVTs remains poorly known, and is currently estimated at 0.5% of all strokes.

It occurs at all ages, with a slight predominance in younger women, due to specific factors such as oral contraceptives, pregnancy and childbirth.

3 DEFINITION:

Cerebral venous thrombosis is a rare form of stroke that results from thrombosis (occlusion due to a blood clot) of the cerebral venous sinus (the main vein draining blood from the brain).

They can cause problems with cerebrospinal fluid evacuation, leading to intracranial hypertension and cerebral lesions such as hemorrhages or infarcts, sometimes in multiple locations. Diagnosis is sometimes difficult. Their prognosis is much better than that of cerebral arterial accidents.

4 ANATOMY :

Cerebral venous thrombosis (CVT) is defined as the more or less complete obstruction of a brain vein. Cerebral veins include the superficial and deep cerebral veins that drain into the venous sinuses of the dura mater (superior longitudinal, inferior longitudinal, right, petrous, sphenoidal and lateral venous sinuses).

The dura mater sinuses drain into the two internal jugular veins.

4.1 CEREBRAL VEINS

Are divided into 3 contingents of different topography and function:

4.1.1 Superficial venous network (cortical veins)

Drains the cerebral cortex and immediately underlying white matter to the superior longitudinal sinus and lateral sinuses. These superficial veins form a highly-developed anastomotic support network, which in some cases explains the paucity of symptoms. Thrombosis of this type of vein may be complicated by localized edema and venous infarction. Cortical veins or superficial cerebral veins include (16) :

1.1.1. A superior group: formed by the ascending frontal, parietal and occipital veins, which drain countercurrently into the superior sagittal sinus (SSS).

1.1.2An anteroinferior group: consisting of the low frontal and insular veins that drain into the cavernous sinus.

These veins are linked by Tolard's great anastomotic vein, which connects the SSS to the internal cerebral veins, which are in turn connected to the SL by Labbé's vein. They have thin walls with no muscular fibers or valves, enabling them to dilate and reverse blood flow when the sinus into which they drain is occluded.

They are anastomosed to each other by a large number of collaterals, allowing, in the event of occlusion, the development of a sinus replacement circulation (appearing on angiography as a corkscrew varicose dilatation) and probably explaining the good prognosis of certain cerebral vein thrombosis (CVT).

The anatomical variability in the number and location of cortical veins, as well as the possibility of flow reversal and the development of collateral circulation, account for the absence of well-defined venous territories and, consequently, of well-defined anatomoclinical syndromes for CVTs(16).

4.1.2 The deep vein network

Ensures venous drainage of the diencephalon, basal ganglia and deepest white matter. It collects in the inferior longitudinal sinus and the right sinus. This deep contingent has no anastomosis. Thrombosis at this level can lead to intracranial hypertension.

The deep cerebral veins consist mainly of the internal cerebral veins (ICV) and the basilar veins (BV):

4.1.2.1 Internal cerebral veins :

Formed by the union of subependymal veins. Each internal cerebral vein arises at the apex of Monro's foramen and travels between the two layers of choroidal tissue of the third ventricle, on the upper surface of the thalamus, describing a curve with anterior and superior convexity. It empties into the ampulla of Galen (or great cerebral vein), which is prolonged by the right sinus. It drains the venous return of the periventricular white matter and the nuclei of the brain.

4.1.2.2 Basilar veins:

They arise on either side of the anterior perforated space. They run backwards, bypassing the lateral surface of the cerebral peduncle, and drain into Galen's ampulla. They drain the medial temporal veins of the temporal horn, the grey nuclei of the thalamus and the cerebral peduncle. Unlike the superficial veins, the deep system is constant and always visualized on angiography, so its occlusion is easily recognized (16).

4.1.3 The venous network draining the posterior fossa

To the jugular veins via Galien's great vein, the right sinus and the lateral sinuses. This network is also rich in anastomoses. Veins of the posterior fossa can be divided into three groups:
- draining into the Galien vein,
- draining into the petrous sinus,
- draining into the torcular or lateral sinuses.

Their course is variable, and diagnosis of occlusion is very difficult (16).

(Voirefig 1)

Figure 1: Anatomy of cerebral veins (phlebo-MRI)
Side view (A) and front view (B)) (17)

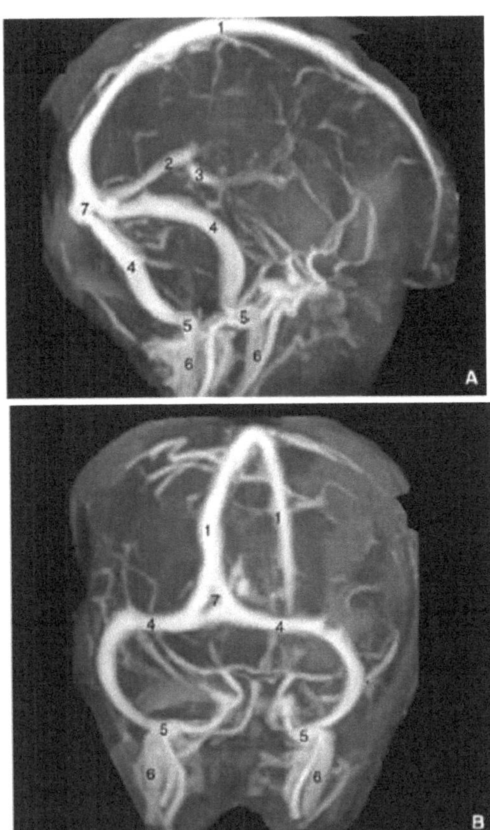

Figure 1. Anatomie des veines cérébrales (phlébo-IRM), vue latérale (A) et antérieure (B). 1. Sinus longitudinal (ou sagittal) supérieur ; 2. sinus droit ; 3. veine de Galien ; 4. sinus latéral (ou transverse) ; 5. sinus sigmoïde ; 6. veine jugulaire interne ; 7. torcular.

4.2   CEREBRAL SINUSES

4.2.1   Median and odd sinuses

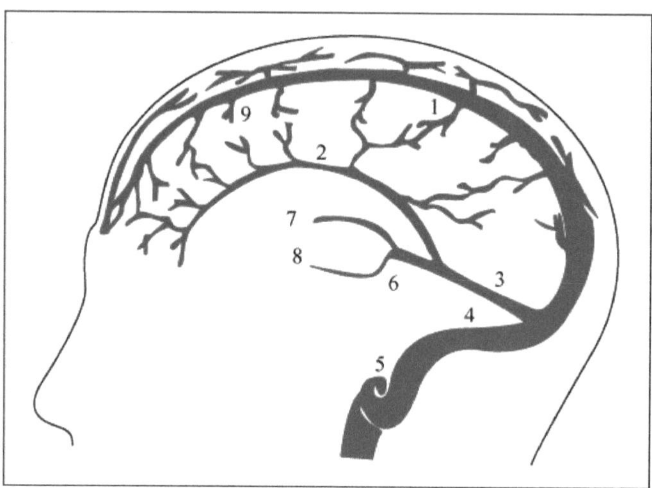

Figure 2:(23). *The cerebral venous system: 1 = superior longitudinal sinus, 2 = inferior longitudinal sinus, 3 = rectus sinus, 4 = transverse sinus, 5 = sigmoid sinus, 6 = Galen's vein, 7 = internal cerebral vein, 8 = basilar vein, 9 = cortical veins.*

4.2.1.1   *Superior sagittal sinus:*

Is a duplication of the dura mater belonging to the brain scythe, opposite the metopic and sagittal suture. It extends from the crista-galli to the Herophilus press. It receives blood from the fronto-ethmoidal vein and cerebral cortex. It drains into the right transverse sinus (13).

The SSS and other sinuses play an important role in cerebrospinal fluid (CSF) circulation, as they communicate laterally via venous lacunae with the arachnoid villi (Pacchioni's granulations), one of the main sites of CSF resorption (13).

There is thus a direct relationship between intracerebral venous pressure and CSF pressure, so that in the event of thrombosis of the SSS or SL, intracranial hypertension frequently occurs (fig 2).

4.2.1.2   Inferior sagittal sinus:

It occupies the posterior 2/3 of the scythe of the brain and empties into the left transverse sinus.

4.2.1.3   Right sinus:

Located at the intersection between the cerebral scythe and the cerebellar tent. It is short and oriented posteroanteriorly, slightly obliquely cephalic. Anteriorly, it receives Galien's veins, the inferior sagittal sinus and the 2 basilar veins; posteriorly, it receives the superior sagittal sinus. It empties into the transverse sinus (13).

4.2.1.4   The occipital sinus:

Runs from the foramen magnum to the internal protuberance of the occiput, inside the cerebellum scythe. It flows into the Herophilus press (13).

4.2.1.5   Circular sinus:

It consists of two cavernous sinuses and surrounds the pituitary gland. It empties into the upper and lower petrous sinuses.

4.2.1.6   The basilar plexus:

Located above the sphenoid and the base of the occiput, it flows into the circular sinus.

4.2.2   Bilateral sinuses

2.2.1. Transverse sinuses:

They follow a groove in the squamous part of the occiput from the Herophilus press towards the posterior torn hole. After crossing the attachment of the cerebellum tenta, they continue their course between the mastoid part of the temporal bone and the jugular part of the occiput as the sigmoid sinus (15) (fig. 2, 3).

4.2.2.1   Cavernous sinuses :

Lateral to the body of the sphenoid. They receive blood from the ophthalmic vein, are drained by the sinuses and constitute the venous confluence between the cerebral veins, the facial veins and the veins of the posterior fossa (13; 15).

They consist of trabeculated cavities separated by different planes of dura mater. Oculomotor nerves III and IV, as well as the ophthalmic and maxillary branches of the trigeminal nerve, pass through the outer wall of the sinus. The external oculomotor nerve (abducens) and the internal carotid artery run inside the sinus.

The cavernous sinus drains blood from the orbits (via the ophthalmic veins) and the anterior part of the brain base (via the sphenoparietal sinuses and middle cerebral veins). The petrous sinuses allow posterior evacuation of the cavernous sinus into the internal jugular veins.

The cavernous sinuses are frequently involved in infections of the face or sphenoidal cavity. Their involvement is therefore usually related to an infectious cause, unlike that of the other sinuses. They are well visualized on MRI or CT, but rarely injected on angiography (13;15).

4.2.2.2   Superior petrosal sinus :

Run along the petrous margin of the temporal bone inside the cerebellum tent, from the cavernous sinuses to the transverse sinuses (13;15).

4.2.2.3   Inferior petrosal sinus:

From the cavernous sinus, they run along the suture of the petro-basilar suture to the anterior part of the posterior tear trough. The SLs drain blood from the cerebellum, brainstem and posterior hemispheres. They also receive some of the diploid veins and venules from the middle ear, which can be a transmission route for a nearby infection (otitis, ENT infection) (17).

There are many anatomical variations in the SL that can lead to misdiagnosis of thrombosis. The right SL, which is wider than the left, is often a direct extension of the SSS. Isolated absence of transverse sinus filling is more suggestive of hypoplasia than thrombosis (13).

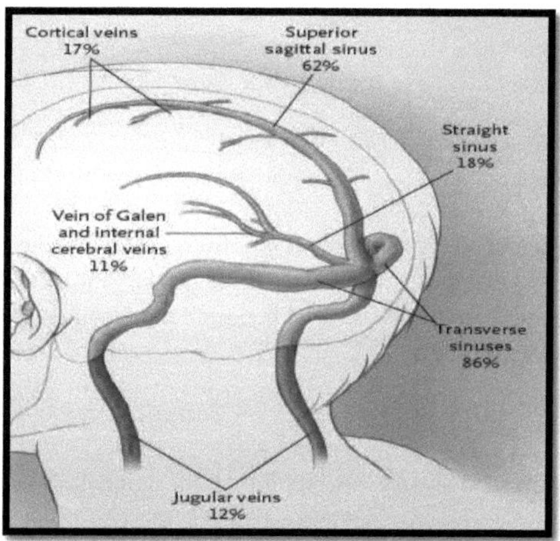

Figure 3: Cerebral sinuses and veins

4.3   ROLES AND CHARACTERISTICS OF CEREBRAL VEINS AND SINUSES

Cranial veins and sinuses are valvular, inelastic, inextensible and non-contractile. Their drainage therefore highlights the presence of a pumping mechanism. This is the primary respiratory movement. Any lesion that limits the expression of cranial respiratory movement has a negative effect on cranial blood drainage.

There is also a pressure-difference suction mechanism during the inspiratory phase. During thoracic inspiration, the pressure of the superior vena cava decreases, causing blood to be drawn from the jugular veins into the right atrium of the heart (13). This means that people who breathe solely through their abdomen potentially lose the benefit of this suction. For this reason, working the thoracic diaphragm will have a positive impact on cranial venous drainage.

As the venous sinuses are in fact a duplication of the cranial dura mater, we can assume that the relaxation of the intracranial membranes has a direct impact on this circulation. The role of these sinuses is not only to transport deoxygenated blood, but also to act as a reserve in case of emergency, especially via the deep venous system. The venous sinuses also play a vital role in fluid balance.

4.4   ROLE IN FLUCTUATING CEPHALO-SPINAL FLUID(13)

Cerebrospinal fluid circulates in the sub-arachnoid space between the maggot (which lines the brain's convolutions) and the arachnoid. It is formed by filtering blood plasma through the choroid plexuses located in the ventricles. CSF enables the elimination of metabolisms harmful to the organism, lymphatic drainage, hormonal transmission, maintenance of homeostasis, and protection of brain matter against shock. CSF pressure is controlled by the secretion/absorption mechanism (fig. 4).

During inspiration, CSF is distributed, while during expiration, arachnoid villi, Pacchioni's granulations, located on the walls of the superior longitudinal venous sinuses1 allow unidirectional passage of CSF to the veins by osmosis or active transport.
The venous sinuses therefore help to maintain the intracranial pressure gradient.

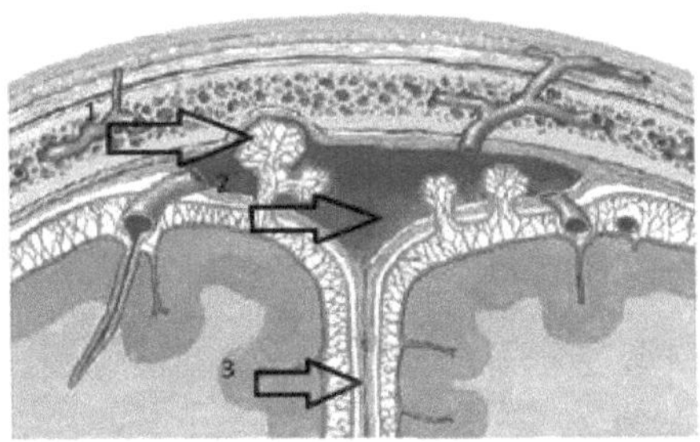

Figure 4 .1 Arachnoid granulations2. Superior longitudinal sinus3. Faulty brain. Role of arachnoid granulations: Resorbs cerebrospinal fluid (cauliflower shape).

4.5   CIRCULATORY MOVEMENTS

4.5.1 1ᵉʳ movement:

Originates in the ophthalmic veins, continues into the cavernous and petrous sinuses, then passes through the posterior foramen magnum and terminates in the internal jugular vein (17) Bone relationships that may influence venous drainage of the first stream: sphenoidal cleft, sphenobasilar symphysis, petrobasilar joint, posterior foramen magnum.

4.5.2 2ᵉᵐᵉ movement:

Originates in Breschet's sphenoparietal sinus, continues in the cavernous sinus to the superior petrous sinus and joins the transverse sinus.

Bone relationships that may influence venous drainage of the second stream: Pteryon, coronal suture, sphenobasilar symphysis, durocher superior medial border, jugular petroleum joint, posterior torn hole

4.5.3 3ᵉᵐᵉ movement:

Originates in the fronto-ethmoidal vein, continues into the superior longitudinal sinus and opens at Herophilus' press. Continues in the right transverse sinus, then in the right sigmoid sinus and ends in the internal jugular vein. Bone relationships that may influence venous drainage of the third stream: ethmoidal notch of the frontal, metopic suture, Bregma, sagittal suture, Lambda, occipital scale, right asterion, right mastoid, right jugular petroleum joint.

4.5.4 4ᵉᵐᵉ movement:

2 origins, Gallien's veins and the inferior longitudinal sinus, leads to the right sinus, then Herophilus' press, then the left sigmoid sinus to the left internal jugular vein. Bone relationships that may influence venous drainage of the fourth stream:

Sagittal suture, inion, left asterion, left mastoid, left jugular petroleum joint.

4.5.5 5th movement:

Origin in the posterior occipital sinus, which opens into the internal jugular vein. Bone relationships that may influence fifth-stream venous drainage: Foramen magnum, petrous jugular joint, posterior torn hole (13) (fig 6).

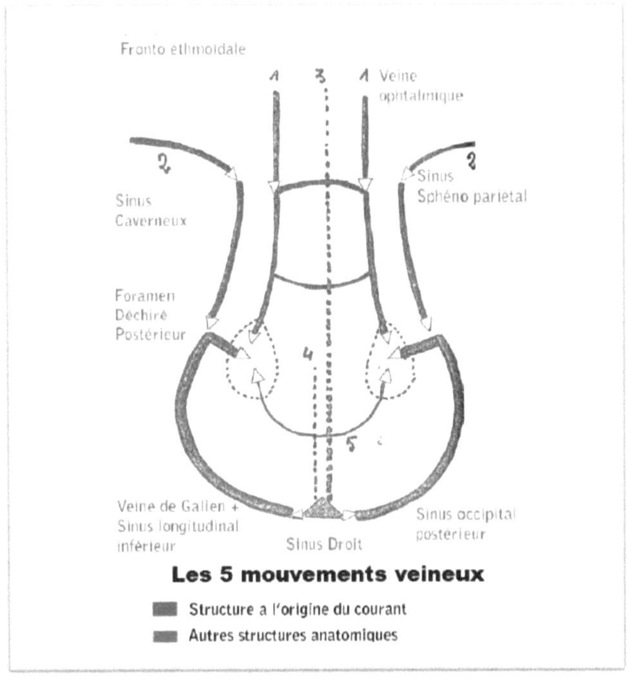

Figure 6: The 5 venous movements(13)

5 PHYSIOLOGY AND PHYSIOPATOLOGY :

The cerebral venous system comprises rigid structures, the dural sinuses, into which deep and cortical veins drain, the latter being of variable topography and thin wall. In the event of a CVT, these cortical veins are frequently dilated or flow reversed, and collateral circulation develops. This possibility of supplementation temporarily helps to limit the severity of brain damage.

Within the sinuses are the arachnoid villi, which drain the cerebrospinal fluid (CSF). CSF normally flows from the ventricles through the subarachnoid spaces towards the base and surface of the brain, to the arachnoid villi, where it is absorbed and drained into the venous sinuses. Sinus thrombosis results in impaired CSF resorption and intracranial hypertension (ICHT).

Cerebral vein obstruction may be complicated by brain parenchymal lesions, sometimes referred to as venous infarction, but essentially comprising vasogenic edema secondary to rupture of the blood-brain barrier by venous stasis. This rupture causes plasma to leak into the interstitial space, resulting in edematous lesions and sometimes local hemorrhage. These lesions vary in size and composition (isolated cerebral edema, "venous" ischemia, simple hemorrhagic petechiae within an edema to voluminous intra-parenchymal hematoma. They may be reversible if the veins are permeabilized, which distinguishes them from lesions secondary to arterial ischemia, where cytotoxic edema precedes cell death. Diffusion sequence

Magnetic resonance imaging (MRI) is useful for assessing the prognosis of parenchymal lesions of venous origin. Hyper signals may or may not be present, and the apparent diffusion coefficient (ADC) of hyper signals may be normal, reduced or increased. In cases of increased ADC (vasogenic edema), tissue lesions generally disappear. They have a better prognosis than cytotoxic edema lesions. Injection-free cerebral CT scan (left) and flair sequence magnetic resonance imaging (right). Cerebral venous thrombosis of the right lateral sinus, edema complicated by hemorrhagic transformation and diminished ADC, which are irreversible (except in the event of a comital crisis). Their distinction explains the better recovery of edematous or hemorrhagic parenchymal lesions of venous origin compared to those of arterial origin.

Anatomical variations in the venous system explain the clinical polymorphism. Involvement of the venous sinuses accounts for the frequency of HTIC even in the absence of parenchymal lesions. Finally, the reversible nature of vasgenic edema (as opposed to cytotoxic edema) contributes to the good prognosis for neurological recovery.

6 CLINICAL ASPECTS

CVTs occur at any age, with an average age of 40 and a slight predominance of younger women, and the mode of onset is subacute (48 hours) in 50% of cases, sudden, sometimes thunderclap-like, in 30% and progressive (more than 30 days) in 20%. *Table I lists* the clinical signs most frequently encountered in CVT.

The clinical symptoms and signs of cerebral venous thrombosis (CVT) are highly varied, and easy evocation of CVT is essential for early diagnosis (4;5).

Classic symptoms and signs (5)

Table 4: Main symptoms and clinical signs of CVT [5].
Headache 85
Papilloedema 47
Focal deficit 42
Convulsive seizures 41
Impaired alertness 29

– Headaches

They are the most frequent clinical symptom, present in 74 to 91% of cases. They have no specific characteristics. They may begin gradually (>24 hours) in 65% of cases, acutely (<24 hours) in 17.5% of cases, or abruptly (<1 minute) in 17.5% of cases.

They may be diffuse or localized, radiating into the cervical region, and range in intensity from a simple feeling of a heavy head to a thunderclap headache suggestive of meningeal hemorrhage, or may mimic a migraine attack whose unusual character (intensity or duration) will attract attention(4).

- **Focal signs, epileptic manifestations, vigilance disorders :**

In 77% of cases, headaches are associated with other neurological symptoms (focal signs, epileptic manifestations, vigilance disorders), and this association rapidly evokes the diagnosis of cerebral venous thrombosis.

Focal signs These may include motor or sensory deficits, language disorders or visual field impairment.

Partial and/or generalized **epileptic seizures** may also occur (10-48% of cases).

These symptoms testify to the suffering of the cerebral parenchyma secondary to impeded venous drainage, which may be responsible for cerebral edema, leading to venous ischemia or cerebral hemorrhage.

The inter-individual variation in cerebral venous anatomy, and the frequent association of thrombosis in several sinuses and veins, make precise clinico-topographic correlation difficult (5), as in arterial cerebral ischemia.

Involvement of the SLS (70%) and SL (70%) is the most frequent, followed by involvement of the right sinus (15%) and cavernous sinus (3%).

The clinical course of cerebral venous thrombosis can be classically summarized as **4 different pictures,** depending on the site of thrombosis and its extension, particularly to the cortical veins:

- **Focal signs** (constituted, transient deficit and/or comitial seizure) isolated or associated with signs of intracranial hypertension, or even vigilance disorders. This is the most frequent presentation;

- Isolated **intracranial hypertension** associated with headache, papilledema and sometimes diplopia due to VI involvement;

- **Diffuse encephalopathy characterized** mainly by psychic disorders, confusion or coma, possibly associated with comitial seizures.

- **Thrombosis of the cavernous sinus** characterized by painful ophthalmology and chemosis homolateral to the thrombosis, exophthalmos as well as sensory disturbances in the innervation zone of the first trigeminal branch to be feared in case of malignant staphylococcal disease of the face.
- **Lemière syndrome** following Fusobacteriumnecrophorum angina or pharyngitis => septic thrombus formation in nearby veins with locoregional extension and septic metastases (notably pulmonary) (23)
These clinical aspects account for the greatest number of cerebral venous thromboses. However, there are also **some unusual features, which** can make the diagnosis difficult to make:

- Transient symptoms such as isolated coma or TIA;
- Psychiatric disorders;
- Symptoms mimicking a migraine with or without aura ;
- Isolated headache.

This picture of headache as the only symptom of cerebral venous thrombosis with a normal CT scan and lumbar puncture was found in 14% of cases in a series of 123 patients, underlining the fact that any recent and unusual headache should be explored urgently in search of CVT (table 5).

Table 5: (6) First symptoms of sinus vein thrombosis

Early clinical symptoms of thrombosis sinus veins
Common symptoms
Isolated intracranial hypertension accompanied by headaches
Focal syndrome (deficit and/or seizures) Diffuse encephalopathy
Any combination of the above
Rare symptoms
Cavernous sinus syndrome
Subarachnoid hemorrhage
Thunderclap headache Migraine attack with aura
Isolated headaches
Transient ischemic attack
Tinnitus
Isolated psychiatric signs Single or multiple cranial nerve deficits

7 RADIOLOGICAL DIAGNOSIS

The diagnosis of CVT is based not only on imaging of the brain parenchyma, but also on vascular imaging, which reveals thrombosis of the cerebral sinuses and/or veins:

7.1   Cerebral computed tomography:(16)

Cerebral CT scans without and with injections are the first examinations to be carried out when CVT is suspected. Although it rarely provides proof of CVT, it remains the most common examination for clearing up the problem, and initially enables us to rule out the many other conditions, such as tumors, abscesses or encephalitis, which can give rise to the same clinical symptoms. These are classified into direct and indirect signs (16).

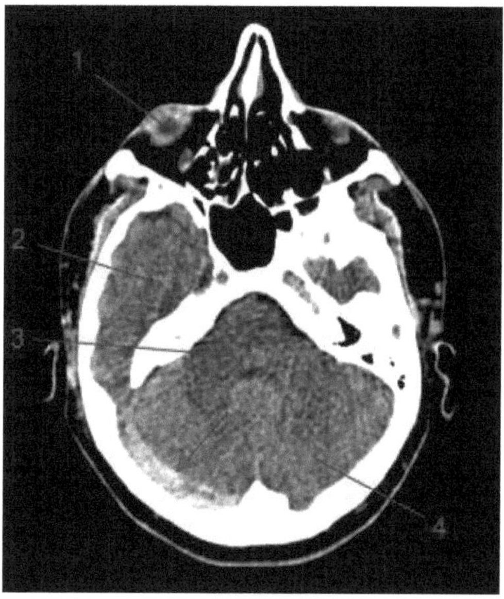

Figure 8. Cerebral CT scan, axial section without intravenous contrast injection. 1, Ocular globe. 2, Right temporal lobe. 3, Fourth ventricle. 4, Cerebellum. Arrow, spontaneously hyperdense right transverse sinus.(26)

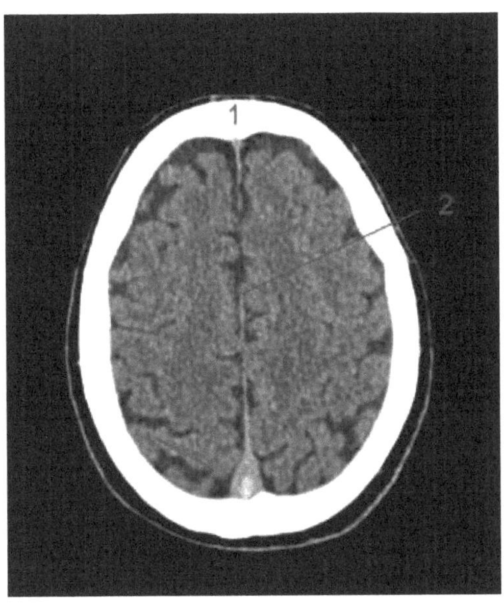

Figure9. Cerebral CT scan, axial section without intravenous contrast injection.1, Frontal pole. 2, False brain. Arrow, The thrombus located in the superior sagittal sinus appears spontaneously and discreetly hyperdense.(26)

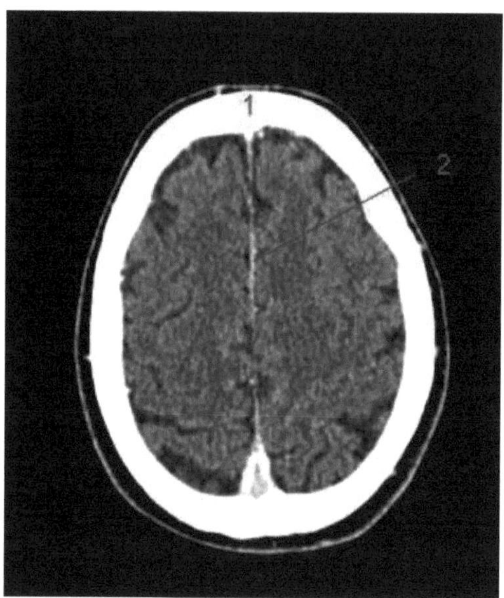

Figure 10. Cerebral CT scan, axial section after intravenous contrast injection.1, Frontal pole. 2, False brain. Arrow, The central part of the sagittal sinus appears much more hypodense than the periphery.(26)

7.1.1   Direct signs of cerebral venous thrombosis

Without injection, the spontaneous hyperdensity of thrombosis is referred to as the "rope sign" when located in a cortical vein, and as the "dense triangle" in the superior sagittal sinus *(16)*.

 This is a very early but rare sign. It has also been described in the lateral and right sinuses. It is sometimes difficult to confirm because of the hyperdense bony environment, the less dense surrounding brain tissue, or in certain clinical situations (high hematocrit, child). On the image with injection, the "delta" or "empty triangle" sign may be found, corresponding to the contrast of the richly vascularized walls of the superior sagittal sinus, contrasting with the non-injection of the thrombosed lumen*(16)*.

This is the most frequent direct sign, present in approximately 20% of published cases. It appears from the fifth day of evolution and disappears after 2 months [16]. Considered to be almost pathognomonic, it can however be simulated by certain rare cases of bifidity of the terminal part of theSSS.

Figure11: SCANNER/DIRECT SIGNS(25)

Signes du triangle dense

Signe de la corde

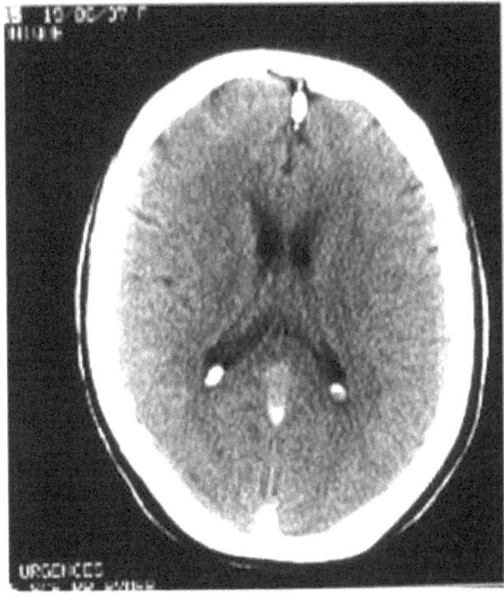

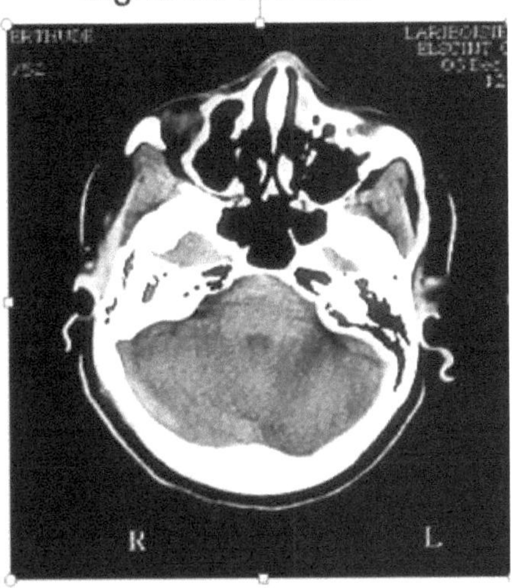

Signe du delta vide (triangle)

• Souvent retardé

• Non constant

• Faux positif
  • division haute du sinus

Figure 12:SCANNER WITH INJECTION(25)

Before injection, clot hyperdensity within a cortical vein or sinus may be visible in the initial stage of thrombosis, but its frequency is rare (< 10%).

After contrast injection, the sinus may take on a so-called empty triangle appearance (delta sign): the sinus lumen appears hypodense, surrounded by increased contrast from the hyperemic sinus walls. This sign often only appears 2 to 3 days after venous occlusion. It is found in 20% of cases of intracranial venous sinus thrombosis.

7.1.2 Indirect signs of venous thrombosis cerebral (19)

These are much more variable than the previous ones and are not very specific. but should attract attention in a clinical context suggestive of cerebral thrombophlebitis .

7.1.2.1 *Cerebral edema*

It may appear diffuse or localized, and is marked by hypodensity of subcortical white matter associated with a mass effect on neighboring structures : compression of ventricular structures or obliteration of hemispheric cortical sulci . When this edema is diffuse , the only abnormality may be a disappearance of the hemispheric cortical sulci and a marked reduction in the size of the ventricles , , which should attract attention , particularly over the age of fifty(19).

7.1.2.2 *Venous softening*

The infarcts are often hemorrhagic, affecting the cortex and white matter . In the infarcted zone, there is frequently a rupture of the blood-brain barrier responsible for contrast uptake. Scanographic findings are highly variable:

a)   **Non-hemorrhagic swelling** :

Relatively frequent, diagnosis is often difficult :

- before injection , it is usual to observe a cortico-subcortical hypodensity accompanied by a mass effect and testifying to a focal cerebral edema .

- after injection , cortical gyriform or nodular subcortical contrast is frequently observed within the hypodense zone .

Finally, edematous hypodensity may be absent and the only visible abnormalities are often very limited gyriform contrast patches .

b)   **Hemorrhagic softening**

They can take several forms: most often, the haemorrhage is discrete (multiple hyperdensities of 1 to 2 cm in diameter within a hypodensity) , sometimes there are voluminous irregular haemorrhagic lesions , peculiar in the immediate presence of an oedematous hypodensity and in their cortico-subcortical topography; they are characteristic when they are multifocal or bilateral (19).

Figure 13 SCANNER/INDIRECTSIGNS(25)

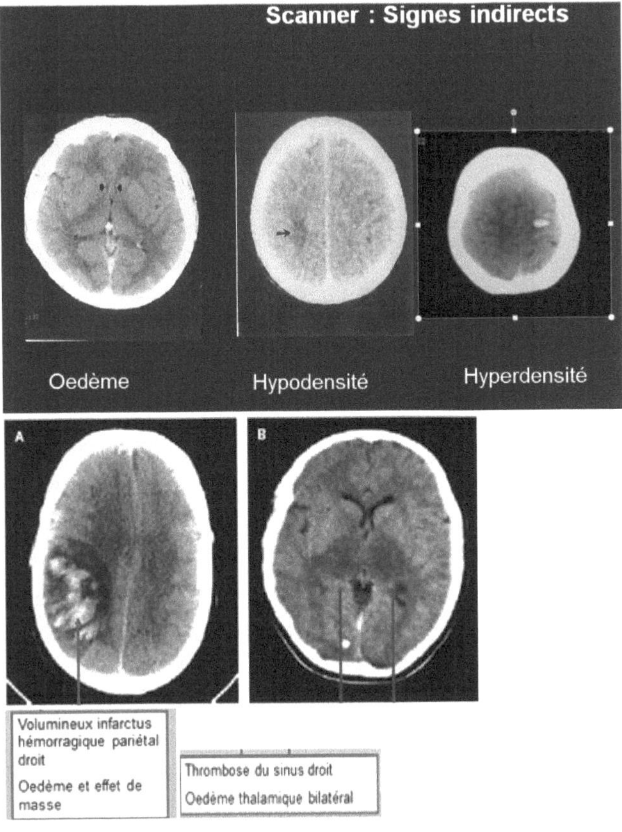

7.2 Magnetic resonance imaging (MRI) :

This imaging technique has two major advantages when it comes to investigating cerebral venous thrombosis: its sensitivity to the speed of flow in the vessels, and the quasi-specificity of the signal given by the products of hemoglobin degradation during thrombosis or hemorrhage. These properties enable us to highlight both vascular occlusion phenomena and their impact on brain tissue.

MRI is the gold standard for diagnosing DVT, as it visualizes thrombosis, its progression and sometimes the underlying cause. It is the non-traumatic method of choice for the study of blood flow, and is therefore ideally suited to the study of thrombophlebitis c ébrale(14).

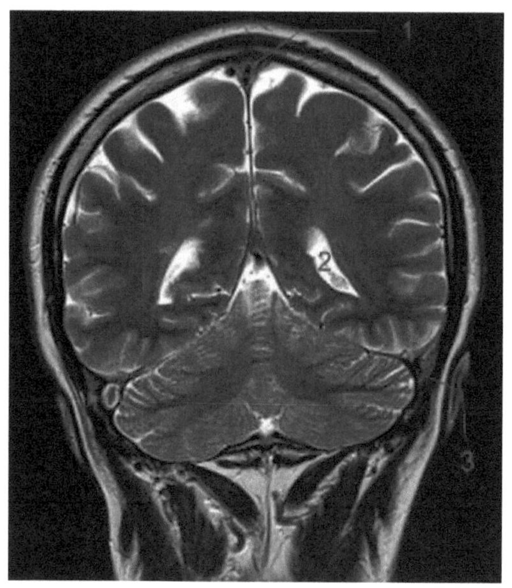

Figure 14. Cerebral MRI, T2 coronal slice. 1, Superior sagittal sinus (heterogeneous signal). 2, Lateral ventricle. 3, Left transverse sinus ("void signal"). Arrow, Thrombosed right transverse sinus.(26)

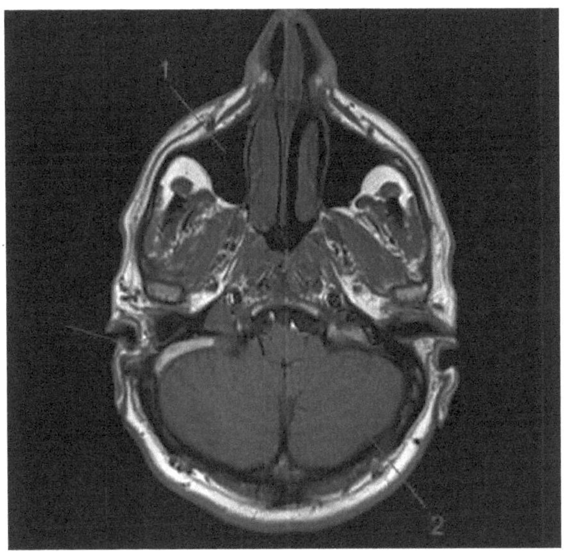

Figure 15. cerebral MRI, T1 axial section.1, Maxillary sinus. 2, Cerebellum. Arrow, Thrombosed sigmoid sinus (26)

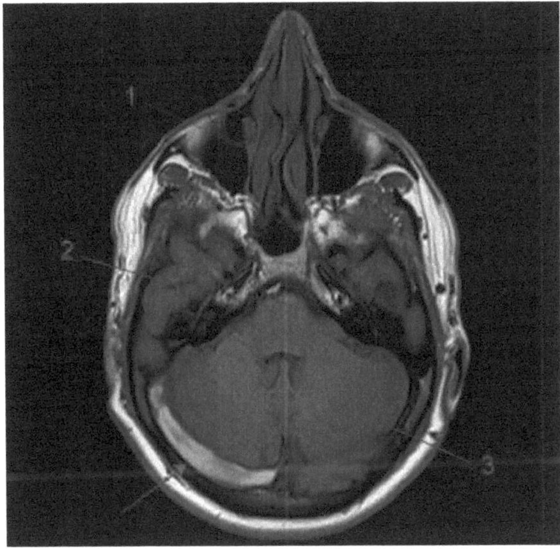

Figure 16. Cerebral MRI, T1 axial slice.1, Right maxillary sinus. 2, Right temporal lobe. 3, Cerebellum. Arrow, Thrombosed right transverse sinus.(26)

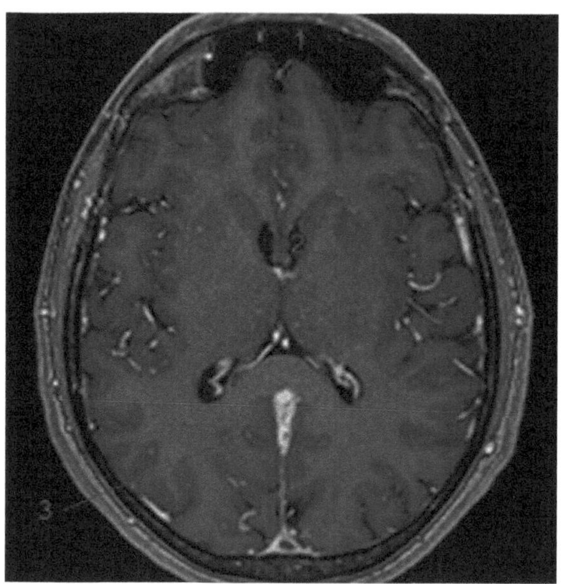

Figure 17. Cerebral MRI, T1 axial slice, after gadolinium. 1, Frontal sinus. 2, Lateral ventricle. 3, Right sinus (heterogeneous appearance). Arrow, The central part of the sagittal sinus appears much more hypodense than the periphery (26).

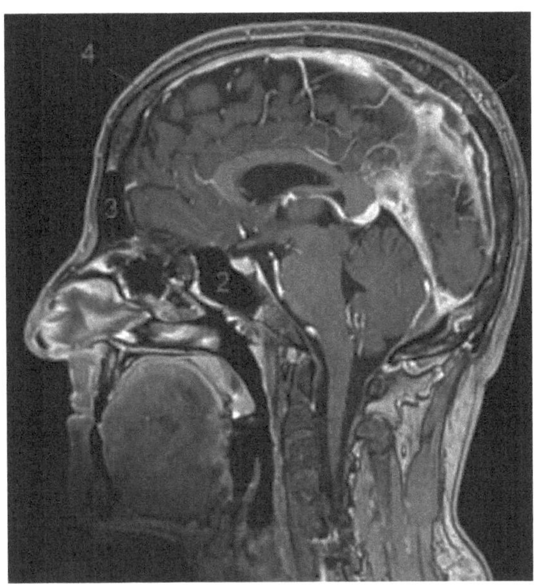

Figure 18. cerebral MRI, T1 sagittal section, after gadolinium.1, Cerebellum. 2, Sphenoidal sinus. 3, Frontal sinus. 4, Corpus callosum. Arrow, Thrombus located in the superior sagittal sinus . Abnormalities concern both thrombosed cerebral veins and the impact of thrombosis on brain tissue . (26)

7.2.1 Occlusion of the dura mater sinuses

Occlusion of the dura mater sinuses results in the appearance of an abnormal signal in the vascular lumen . On T1 , in the first few days the sinus loses its hypo flow signal and becomes iso signal, then from the fourth day, after the onset of venous thrombosis , it appears hyper signal, indicating the presence of extracellular methemoglobin. Shortly afterwards, the thrombus also appears as a T2-weighted hyper signal .

Beyond the third week, after the onset of venous thrombosis , the T1-weighted hyper signal disappears, while T2-weighted signal abnormalities remain visible as long as venous thrombosis persists . Unfortunately, flow artifacts can give rise to hyper signals(14) simulating thrombosis . A hyper signal in a sinus must be seen in both planes to be considered pathological. On the other hand , in the very early days (deoxyhaemoglobin stage), the thrombus may be hyposignal on all sequences, simulating a permeable sinus.

Angio-MRI is a very useful complement to MRI in the exploration of sinus thrombosis by demonstrating the absence of flow in occluded veins .

In many cases, these two complementary procedures can be used to diagnose cerebral venous thrombosis , but there are limitations (14). These may be related to the patient's state of agitation, particularly at the acute stage, which may make MRI or angiomicrography impractical, or to the highly localized nature of the occlusion or the small size of the veins affected , particularly in purely cortical thrombosis .

7.2.2 Venous infarctions

On MRI, they appear as oval or rounded cortico-subcortical lesions , very edematous and often hemorrhagic : in T1-weighted sequence , the lesions are moderately hypo-signal, associated in 80% of cases with hyper-signal areas associated with hemorrhagic remodeling . In T2-weighted sequences, venous infarcts appear as a hyper-signal corresponding to cerebral edema, within which there is frequently a more pronounced hyper-signal zone , bordered by a thin hypo-signal border corresponding to the area of hemorrhage (14).

It shows the absence of opacification of venous structures and enables precise assessment of lesion extension and recanalization. The limitations of this technique are the study of cortical veins and segmental thrombosis.

Magnetic resonance angiography: This now usually replaces conventional angiography. Several techniques are used: time-of-flight or phase contrast. The diagnosis of thrombosis is made in the absence of flow. It can be particularly useful in cases of "false negatives" on MRI, particularly in the early phase, or in cases of "false positives" linked to the presence of slow flows that appear as a hyper signal on MRI. MRA can sometimes be difficult to interpret in cases of partial thrombosis, cavernous sinus thrombosis or cortical vein thrombosis.

7.3   Angioscanner :

A diagnostic alternative to the MRI-MRA combination is cerebral angioscan. Easily performed immediately after the CT scan, it shows that the thrombosed sinus is not visible. Certain signs are also suggestive, such as strong contrast of the sinus wall or the presence of collateral circulation (16).

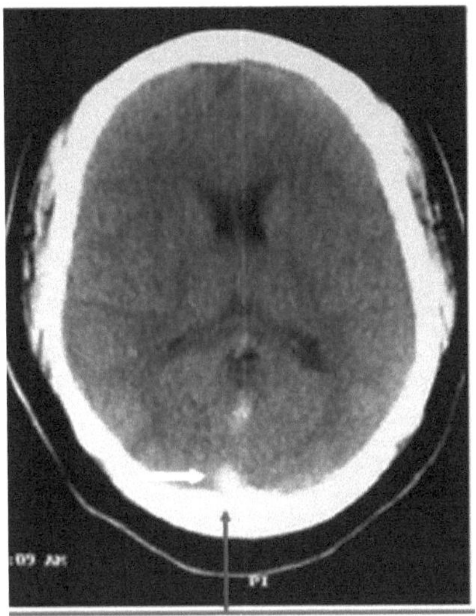

Figure 19:(25) Hyperdensity on injection-free CT scan

7.4   Angiography :

The indications for angiography in the diagnosis of cerebral venous thrombosis have clearly diminished since the advent of MRI . When performed , angiography must be technically perfect, with front , profile and æ views and very late times, often beyond 20ème seconds. Indications for angiography are limited to technical impossibilities, and the shortcomings or contraindications of MRI .

It will reveal three fundamental signs (16): circulatory delay, venous occlusions and bypass routes .

- **Circulatory delay**: very frequent, marked by stagnation of the contrast medium in the cerebral veins , upstream of the occlusion.

-**Venous occlusions** can affect cortical veins , dural sinuses or deep veins . They are more or less easy to detect depending on their location and extension . They correspond to an absence of more or less focused opacification .

- **Suppletive pathways**: sinus or cortical vein occlusion leads to varying degrees of dilatation of a collateral suppletive network : this may involve cortical veins, which take on an irregular, corkscrew appearance , trans-cerebral anastomoses or extra-cerebral (meningeal or even superficial) anastomoses (19.16).

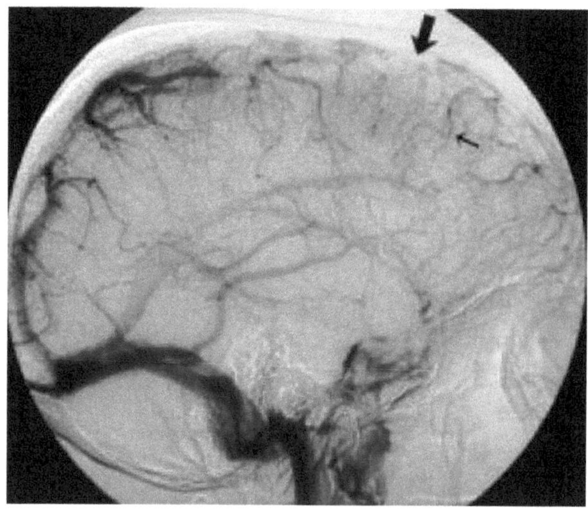

Figure 20 (16) Conventional angiography: extensive occlusion of the superior sagittal sinus (Arrow), corkscrew appearance of collateral veins (small arrow).

The diagnosis of cerebral venous thrombosis should be made on the basis of scannographic signs and clinical data, and confirmed by MRI, if possible in conjunction with angiography . In cases where this confirmation cannot be obtained by MRI , angiography remains necessary to make the diagnosis .

In the absence of a definitive image from the preceding investigations, angiography is sometimes indispensable. This is particularly true in the case of cortical vein thrombosis, sometimes suspected only by the presence of "corkscrew" collateral veins. Angiography must be rigorous: study of all four axes, at least two different views, and if possible a three-quarter view to visualize the entire SSS. Late films are also useful in the absence of opacification of the venous network.

Angiography shows the absence of opacification of thrombosed sinuses and the possible development of collateral circulation. Diagnosis is easy when the interruption is extensive. It can be difficult when the occlusion is localized over 1 to 2 cm, especially as it must be distinguished from a filling defect linked to a washout flow opposite the afference of contralateral cortical veins.

Contralateral angiography can avoid these false positives. Lack of opacification of the transverse portion of the lateral sinuses is sometimes a diagnostic problem, as hypoplasia is common (19;16).

Thrombosis is classically evoked by two signs

- the presence on the skull X-ray of the bone groove corresponding to the occluded lateral sinus;

- visibility of the initial portion of the lateral sinus and/or its abrupt termination.

This differentiation is now most often made on MRI parenchymal slices (T1 sagittal slices). These show the cross-sectional size of the lateral sinus and the presence of any thrombus in the form of a hyper-signal.

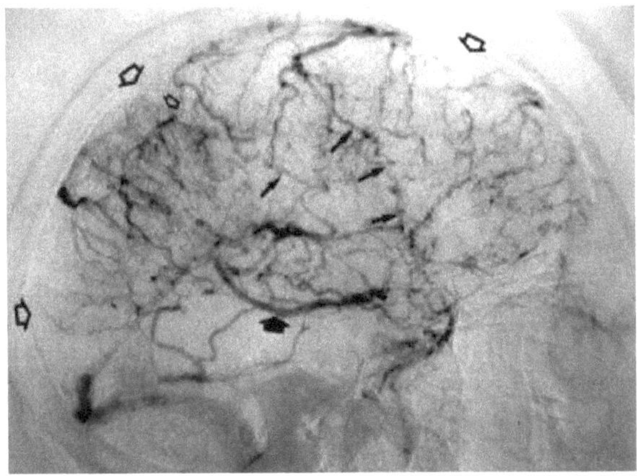

Figure 21 (3). Right internal carotid angiogram. Profile view.1: large empty arrows: non-visualization of the SLS; 2: solid arrow: dilation of Rosenthal's vein; 3: small empty arrow: thrombosis of a cortical vein; 4: black arrows: dilatedortuous veins.

8 Other tests :

8.1   Blood tests

They are not of interest for positive diagnosis. They are important for etiological diagnosis, their disruption pointing to infectious, inflammatory or malignant causes.

A detailed haemostasis work-up should be carried out in the presence of any CVT, as associated causes or favouring factors are frequent. CBC/platelets (check for haemopathy),(6)

Thrombophilia work-up: protein C, protein S, factor V Leyden, antithrombin III, prothrombin G20210A mutation, search for circulating anticoagulant, antiB2GP1, anticardiolipids, antiphospholipids, antinuclear factor(6)

8.2   The benefits of D-dimer measurement

These were most often elevated (>500ng/ml) when the diagnosis of cerebral venous thrombosis was confirmed, with the exception of patients whose symptoms had been evolving for more than 3 weeks(2).

Normal dimers do not exclude the diagnosis of cerebral venous thrombosis. However, they do not reliably rule out this diagnosis, particularly in the face of atypical symptomatologies.

The value of D-dimers in the diagnosis of CVT has not been established. In our personal experience, D-dimers are elevated in most cases of recent DVT, but can sometimes be negative, particularly when symptoms have been evolving for more than 1 month. While the negative predictive value of D-dimers in lower-limb venous thrombosis is well established, it remains to be determined in DVT(2).

8.3   Lumbar puncture,

Often abnormal, showing increased pressure, red or white blood cells and hyperproteinorachia. Cerebrospinal fluid composition and pressure are strictly normal in 10% of cases.

Compositional abnormalities include hyperproteinorachia (rarely greater than 1g/L), an increase in red blood cells above 20/mm3 in two-thirds of cases and/or pleocytosis of variable formula, predominantly mixed lymphocytic or more rarely polynucleated (one-third of cases). The combination of these three anomalies is a classic formula found in 30-50% of cases reported in the literature.

CSF studies are essential in the presence of isolated ICH: for diagnostic purposes, by measuring opening pressure, but also for therapeutic purposes, to rapidly relieve ICH threatening the optic nerves. CSF studies are also useful in febrile forms to rule out meningitis, and in forms with no apparent cause to look for chronic meningitis(16).

8.4   Electroencephalogram :

It is abnormal in around 75% of cases, and shows abnormalities that are often more diffuse than the clinic would suggest, but without any specificity: slowing of the basic rhythm, slow waves in focus, epileptic activity. It is mainly of interest in forms where confusional or psychiatric symptoms predominate(16).

8.5   Venous Doppler (16) :

Currently has a limited role in the diagnosis of DVT.

The state of venous circulation was studied using transcranial Doppler and transcranial ultrasonography. In the case of SSS thrombosis, high velocities were recorded in the deep venous system. Similarly, microembolic signals were recorded in the internal jugular veins. Transcranial Doppler may be useful for close monitoring of extensive SSS thrombosis, enabling daily monitoring.

9 TOPOGRAPHICAL DIAGNOSIS

Signs and symptoms may vary according to the topography of the venous thrombosis. However, the inter-individual variation in cerebral venous anatomy and the frequent association of thrombosis in several sinuses and veins make precise clinicotopographic correlation difficult, as in cerebral arterial ischemia.

Involvement of the SLS (70%) and SL (70%) is the most frequent, followed by involvement of the right sinus (15%) and cavernous sinus (3%)(18).

Thrombosis of the SLS and/or SL is often accompanied by a variable combination of symptoms and signs of intracranial hypertension, focal neurological deficit and seizures(18).

The diagnosis of cavernous sinus thrombosis should be made in the presence of a variable combination of the following signs: chemosis, painful ophthalmoplegia, exophthalmos, palpebral edema, cranial nerve damage (II, III, V1, V2, VI).

Isolated involvement of the VI is possible. Initially unilateral signs and symptoms may become bilateral if thrombosis extends to the contralateral cavernous sinus or other dural sinuses (18).

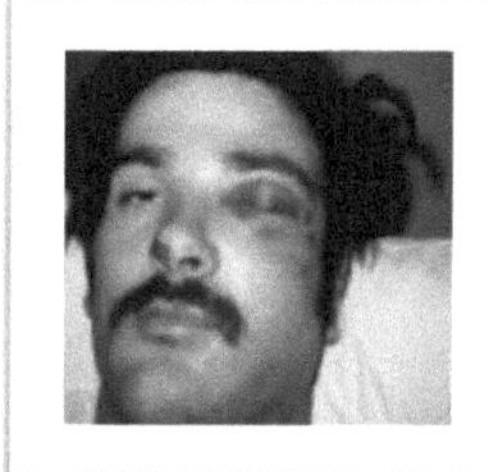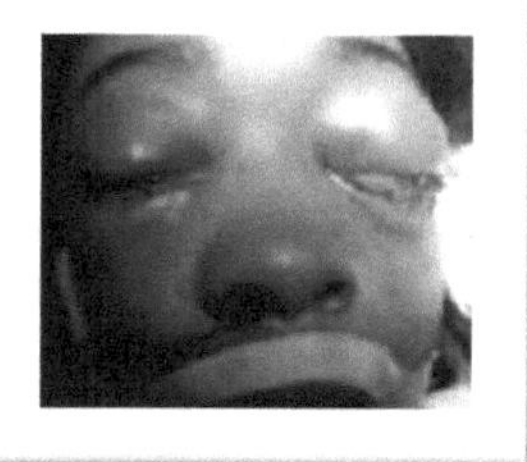

Figure 7: Thrombosis of the cavernous sinus

In the case of deep vein thrombosis, the initial picture is one of consciousness disorders (up to coma) and long tract involvement.

The prognosis is usually severe, with early death or severe sequelae such as akinetic mutism, dementia, bilateral athetoid movements, verticality paralysis and dystonia. Some patients, however, recover satisfactorily. In these cases, the initial picture is less spectacular (neuropsychological disorders sometimes masked by consciousness disorders) and thrombosis is often limited.

Isolated cortical venous thrombosis manifests as seizures and/or focal neurological deficit. Headaches are frequent, with no other signs of intracranial hypertension. Signs tend to fluctuate over the first few days or weeks. Cerebellar venous thrombosis may simulate a posterior fossa tumor.

10   ETIOLOGIES AND RISK FACTORS FOR CTV

10.1   Etiologies of DVT: Table 1

In principle, a distinction is made between infectious (or septic) and non-infectious (or non-septic) forms of cerebral venous thrombosis. Since the widespread availability of antibiotic treatments, the frequency of infectious cerebral venous thrombosis has fallen sharply, at least in industrialized nations (5).

According to large-scale studies, only 6 to 12% of CVTs still have an infectious origin. This is particularly true in children. Both systemic and local infection play a role from a pathophysiological point of view.

Otitis and mastoiditis can lead to cerebral venous thrombosis by continuity, as can infection of the ethmoidal and sphenoidal sinuses, which can typically lead to thrombosis of the cavernous sinus (11).

The list of risk factors for non-infectious cerebral venous thrombosis is long. The etiology of cerebral venous thrombosis is not determined in 15% of patients.

In addition to the known factors that favor deep vein thrombosis of the lower limb, cerebral venous thrombosis can be caused by congenital and acquired disorders of hemostasis, hematological diseases, cancers, connective tissue diseases, vasculitides, metabolic disorders, pregnancy and bed rest (12).

Events that are generally conducive to venous stasis (heart failure, COPD, etc.), as well as local factors (e.g. tumors, arteriovenous malformations, dural fistulas), can favor the onset of CVT. Exogenous factors such as drugs, intoxication and trauma have been described as causes of CVT (5).

Table 1: Causes of sinus vein thrombosis(5)

1. Factors predisposing to venous thrombosis non-infectious brain
Idiopathic (around 15%)
Pregnancy
Postpartum

Exogenous
 Medicines
   - Hormone replacement therapy
   - Oral contraceptives
   - Androgens
   - Chemotherapy
   - Erythropoietin
   - Corticoids
   - Clomipramine
   - Acetazolamide

Poisoning
- Lead
- Carbon monoxide
- Drugs
- Ecstasy

Trauma/intervention
- Craniocerebral trauma
- Brain surgery
- Lumbar puncture, spinal anesthesia, myelography

Hemostasis
- APC resistance (factor V Leiden mutation)
- Protein C, protein S, AT-III deficiency
- Hyperhomocysteinemia
- Anti-phospholipid antibody syndrome
- Disseminated intravascular coagulation
- Heparin-induced type II thrombocytopenia
- Dysfibrinogenemia, plasminogen deficiency
- Prothrombin gene variant
- Paroxysmal nocturnal hemoglobinuria
- Sickle cell anemia, thalassemia
- Bone marrow transplantation
- Thrombocythemia
- Polycythemia vera
- Lymphomas and leukemias
- Monoclonal (Para-)neoplastic gammapathies
- Hypercoagulability
- Carcinomatous meningitis

System disease
- Lupus erythematosus
- Sjögren's syndrome
- Wegener's granulomatosis
- Sarcoidosis
- Behçet's disease (vascular form)

Nephrotoxic syndrome

Flow obstruction and stasis
- Intracranial hypertension
- Mountain sickness
- CSF insufficiency syndrome
- Strangulation
- Malignant tumor
- Meridian dural arteriovenous fistula and arteriovenous

| malformations |
| - Venous catheter |
| - Heart failure, cardiomyopathy |
| - Chronic obstructive pulmonary disease |
| - Morbid adiposity |
| - Severe dehydration |
| - Immobilization |
| **Metabolism** |
| - Thyrotoxicosis |
| - Diabetes |
| - Uremia |
| - Hyperlipidemia |
| **Gastrointestinal diseases** |
| - Ulcerative colitis |
| - Crohn's disease |
| - Cirrhosis of the liver |
| **Local** |
| - Mechanical obstruction to flow, for example, tumor |
| - Arachnoid cyst |
| **2. Cause of cerebral venous thrombosis of infectious origin** |
| **Generalized infection** |
| - Bacterial: septicemia, endocarditis, typhus, tuberculosis |
| - Viral: hepatitis, measles, encephalitis (vhs, hiv), cytomegalovirus |
| - Fungus: aspergillosis |
| - Parasitic: malaria, trichinosis |
| **Local infection** |
| - Mediofacial staphylococcus aureus infection |
| - Otitis, tonsillitis, sinusitis |
| - Stomatitis, dental abscess |
| - Brain abscess, empyema, meningitis |

10.2 Mechanisms and risk factors for cerebral venous thrombosis (Table 2)

10.2.1 Blood stasis

Stasis is a key factor in venous thrombogenesis. On the one hand, it favors the accumulation of various pro-coagulant factors, and on the other, it limits the elimination of activated factors. Various phenomena may be responsible for slowing blood flow (12).

10.2.2 Immobilization

Slows venous return due to lack of muscle contraction. Reduced walking ability due to bedridden conditions or functional impotence is a proven risk factor for postoperative venous thrombosis.

Of course, the occurrence of a thrombotic event is also linked to the type of surgical procedure, the duration of the operation, the underlying pathology or the patient's condition, which may aggravate stasis. Obesity, with its reduced mobility and fibrinolytic activity, could increase the risk of postoperative DVT(12).

10.2.3 Extrinsic compression

(hematoma, cyst, tumor, etc.) or persistent post-thrombotic sequelae, which impede venous return, increase thrombotic risk.

10.2.4 Blood hyperviscosity

In cases of hypercytosis (polycythemia, hyperleukocytosis, leukemia...), dysglobulinemia (myeloma, Waldenström...) is an element not to be neglected.

10.2.5 Dehydration

May reinforce potential plasma hypercoagulability through hemoconcentration of pro-coagulant factors. Diuretics used during congestive heart failure may thus contribute to increasing thrombotic risk by increasing the hemoconcentration associated with blood stasis.

10.2.6 Venous dilatation:

Varicose veins are common, and may increase the risk of thrombosis in the postoperative surgical context, in the event of pregnancy or when taking oestroprogestogenic oral contraception(5) .

10.2.7 Endothelial lesions

The healthy endothelial lining is thermoresistant, thanks to the synthesis of anti-thrombotic substances such as prostacyclin, thrombomodulin, tPA (tissue plasminogen activator) and glycosaminoglycans. The hemostatic balance is nevertheless ensured by the secretion of pro-coagulant factors:

Tissue factor, PAI-1 (tissue plasminogen activator inhibitor), Willebrand factor. Endothelial cells also possess numerous adhesive molecules, ensuring intercellular interactions such as leukoplakellar or leukoendothelial adhesion (E-selectin, VCAM-1, ICAM-1) (12).

They secrete a range of pro-inflammatory cytokines (IL1, IL8, TNF alpha, etc.), helping to amplify cellular activation within the vascular compartment and thus reinforce the procoagulant profile in the event of vascular injury.

There are many causes of endothelial damage:

> surgical trauma:

hip and knee replacement surgery are particularly associated with an increased incidence of phlebitis. Vascular traction and spinal cord trauma are responsible for activating coagulation, leading to high thrombin generation;

> serotherapy
> Venous catheters
> pacemaker lead placement :
> multiple injections by drug addicts
> history of venous thrombosis: relative risk of recurrence

Fivefold increase in case of previous thrombotic episode.

Familial thrombophilia is related to increased thrombin generation in cases of physiological inhibitor deficiency (antithrombin, protein C, protein S) or hypo-fibrinolysis (excess of PAI-1, tPA defect).

It is found in 10-15% of patients with a history of DVT. Resistance to the anticoagulant activity of activated protein C (factor V Leiden), discovered in 1993, and the G20210A mutation in the prothrombin gene, identified in 1996, represent the most frequent constitutional causes (30-50% of patients).

10.2.8 Acquired hypercoagulability(Table2)

The search for pathologies known to be associated with an increased thrombotic risk is extended on the basis of the clinicobiological history. Confirmation of an underlying condition conditions patient management, with etiological treatment combined with anticoagulant therapy. Recently, in the SIRIUS study, Samama et al showed that symptomatic patients had more than one risk factor compared with the control group (1.7 ± 0.05 versus 0.78 ± 0.03), and that the majority of these patients in fact had more than two identified risk factors. These various factors are, on the one hand, specific to the subject and his or her terrain (intrinsic factors), and on the other, linked to a favourable circumstance (extrinsic factors).

Table 2 (11): Relative risks of venous thrombosis induced by factors
Acquired hypercoagulability

Acquired thrombophilia	Relative risk
Age	2,0
Obesity	1,5 à 2,0
History of venous thrombosis	3,0
Cancer	3,07
Surgery	3,0 à 6,0

Estrogen-progestin contraception	4,0 à 6,0
Hormone replacement therapy	2,0
Pregnancy	4,0
Postpartum	14,0
Prolonged immobilization	11,0
Antiphospholipid syndrome	9,0
Congestive heart failure	2,0
Infection	2,5
Varicose veins	2,5

10.2.9 Age

The risk of thrombosis increases dramatically with age, from 1/10,000 before age 40 to 1/1,000 after age 40 and 1/100 over age 75. There is an exponential increase in the risk of venous thrombotic events with advancing age, and several mechanisms are proposed: limited physical mobility, increased blood stasis, co-morbidity (cancer, chronic inflammation, etc.), increased levels of factor VIII, fibrinogen, etc.

10.2.10 Cancers

Cancer is diagnosed in 10-20% of patients with DVT. The onset of an apparently idiopathic thrombotic episode may precede the actual diagnosis of progressive neoplasia by several years]. It is also likely that aggressive treatments (cytolytic chemotherapy, extensive surgery, radiotherapy, etc.) and reduced patient mobility aggravate this acquired thrombophilia. The most thrombogenic cancers are adenocarcinomas of the pancreas, stomach, colon, bladder and ovary.

10.2.11 Hemopathy

Various haemopathies are particularly associated with venous thrombotic risk. These are mainly clonal cell proliferation with chronic myeloproliferative syndromes (< 10% of patients) and lymphoid hemopathies such as Hodgkin's disease or non-Hodgkin's lymphoma. In addition to the standard haemostasis work-up, the search for spontaneous sprouting of haematopoietic progeny is part of the etiological work-up for portal or splanchnic venous thrombosis.

10.2.12 Surgery and trauma

Surgical procedures and severe trauma favor the onset of DVT, and the associated bed rest aggravates blood stasis. Orthopedic surgery and neurosurgery are particularly high-risk situations.

10.2.13 Prolonged immobilization

Strict bed rest is a recognized risk factor for venous thromboembolism. Various situations associated with reduced mobility are also potential triggers. For example, functional impotence or paralysis, wearing a cast, prolonged air travel (over 4 hours) and even heavy city traffic jams can all contribute to thrombus formation.

The first case of DVT associated with estrogen-progestin use was published in 1961, and since then numerous studies have confirmed the increased thrombotic risk. Reducing the ethinylestradiol content (from 100 to 30 µg) significantly reduced this risk, but did not eliminate it. This risk also seems to be linked to the progestins used. Third-generation pills containing desogestrel or gestodene are associated with a higher relative risk of DVT than second-generation pills containing levonorgestrel (RR ' 2). This effect may be partly correlated with the induction of resistance to the anticoagulant activity of activated protein C. But there are also other abnormalities in haemostasis: genuine hypercoagulability due to increased levels of factors VII, X and XII, combined with a reduction in physiological inhibitors such as antithrombin or protein S; and hyperfibrinolysis due to a combination of increased plasminogen and reduced PAI-1 .

10.2.15   Pregnancy and post-scent (Table3)

The prevalence of DVT is around 0.5/1,000 during pregnancy. In women under 40, half of all venous thromboembolic events are related to pregnancy or the postpartum period. Several mechanisms contribute to this increase in thrombotic risk: slower blood flow, reduced venous tone, obstruction of venous return by the gravid uterus, and changes in hemostasis generating a hypercoagulable profile. These disturbances normalize within 6 to 8 weeks of delivery. Optimal management of venous thrombosis during pregnancy is therefore essential. While thrombotic events during pregnancy have important characteristics (90% of cases occur in the left lower limb, mainly at the iliofemoral level, with a high risk of embolization), there is no evidence of a particularly high incidence in any of the trimesters. Overall, two-thirds of thrombotic episodes occur in the post-partum period(5;11;12).

In fact, an association with constitutional thrombophilia should be sought. For example, one study showed that 60% of pregnant women with DVT were carriers of factor V leiden. Apart from the existence of hereditary thrombophilia, thrombotic risk increases with a history of phlebitis, age, multiparity, suppression of lactation by estrogens or caesarean section. In vitro fertilization is a special case, where thrombotic episodes may occur within 2 to 8 weeks of pregnancy induction, preferentially affecting the superior vena cava.

Table 3: Changes in haemostasis during pregnancy(12) .

COAGULATION	FIBRINOLYSIS
↑• Factors VIII, VII, X, X, XII, II, fibrinogen ↓• Antithrombin, Protein S ↑• Protein C, TFPI ↑• Thrombin-Antithrombin complexes, ↑• Prothrombin fragments 1 + 2 ↑• Fibrinopeptides A = **HYPERCOAGULABILITY**	↑• Plasminogen ↑• PAI-1 (and placental PAI- ↓2) • tPA↑ ↑• Ddimers (fibrin formation) ↓• overall fibrinolytic activity = **HYPOFIBRINOLYSIS**

TFPI: tissue factor pathway inhibitor.

tPA: tissue plasminogen activator;

PAI: plasminogen activator inhibitor.

10.2.16   Anti-phospholipid syndrome

A circulating anticoagulant (CCA) of the lupus or antiprothrombinase type is found in around 5% to 15% of patients with DVT. This CCA is also associated with a five- to nine-fold increased thrombotic risk. Certain so-called systemic diseases should also be considered in the context of venous thromboembolic disease: systemic lupus erythematosus (5-20% of cases) and Behçet's disease (10-45% of cases).

Involvement of the large venous trunks is frequent. In ulcerative colitis such as Crohn's disease and ulcerative colitis, the risk of thrombosis is two to three times higher than in the general population (12). Hypercoagulability is thought to be linked, on the one hand, to elevated levels of factor VIII and hyperfibrinogenemia and, on the other, to endothelial damage responsible for tissue factor release, increased cell adhesiveness and elevated levels of factor Willebrand. These abnormalities are not specific.

10.2.17   Iatrogenic or drug-induced venous thrombosis

We have already considered the case of chemotherapy, which is toxic to the endothelium, and estrogen-progestin contraception, which is responsible for genuine systemic hypercoagulability.

Anti-estrogens such as tamoxifen can increase the risk of venous thrombosis. Heparin-induced thrombocytopenia, characterized by a rapid drop in platelet count and the onset of extensive venous thrombotic events, should not be overlooked. This complex syndrome is a rare complication (3 to 5% of treatments with unfractionated heparin and 0.1% of treatments with low-molecular-weight heparin), but a formidable one, with severe morbidity and mortality linked to late and difficult diagnosis.

Nephrotic syndrome, responsible for acquired hypercoagulability through renal leakage of antithrombin, can complicate DVT in adults, but this is much rarer in children.

Erysipelas with lymphangitis is a differential diagnosis of DVT, but may favour the development of genuine thrombosis. Lumière syndrome associates thrombophlebitis of the internal jugular vein and/or pulmonary embolism secondary to Fusobacteriumnecrophorum infection (12).

Thrombosis of the suprahepatic or portal veins is particularly common in paroxysmal nocturnal hemoglobinuria.

11   DIFFERENTIAL DIAGNOSIS OF CTV

The differential diagnosis includes meningitis, encephalitis (eg. The differential diagnosis includes meningitis, encephalitis (e.g. herpetic encephalitis, encephalitis with septic focus), cerebral abscess, cerebral hemorrhage (subdural hematoma, subarachnoid hemorrhage, primary intracerebral hemorrhage), ischemic infarction, cerebral tumor, cerebral edema, as well as benign intracranial hypertension, migraine with and without aura, hypertensive encephalopathy, eclampsia and psychiatric diseases (21).

All pathologies with signs of intracranial hypertension can mimic a CVT. Benign intracranial hypertension should be considered, especially in young women. Encephalitis, meningitis or abscesses can cause signs of intracranial hypertension, but usually in a febrile context.

The various brain tumors can manifest as headaches, seizures and papilledema. Ultimately, clinical examination cannot rule out arterial occlusion or cerebral hemorrhage. In the case of a pauci- or mono-symptomatic presentation, the range of differential diagnoses corresponds to all the pathologies usually considered in the presence of the given symptom (headache, focal neurological deficit or comitial seizure).

The diagnosis of CVT is based on the visualization of thrombus and venous occlusion using neuroimaging techniques (CT or MRI) (21).

12   THERAPEUTIC MANAGEMENT :

The variability of the clinical presentation and the small number of cases mean that treatment cannot be systematized. Nevertheless, it is based on 3 modalities.

12.1   Etiological treatment :

Whenever possible, this is particularly important in septic forms. Specific treatment may also be required for certain general illnesses (cancer, haemopathy, systemic diseases).

In the case of septic CPT, treatment of the infectious site is essential, and relies on antibiotic therapy, sometimes combined with surgical treatment (drainage of maxillary sinusitis, mastoiditis, etc.).

The combination of a 3rd generation cephalosporin (cefotaxime or ceftriaxone) and a product active on anaerobic germs, can be used when the suspected germs arestreptococci and/or anaerobes (20).

Suspicion of S. *aureus* infection (facial or scalp infection, cavernous sinus thrombosis) prompts the prescription of penicillin M . In the case of CPT complicating malignant staphylococcal disease of the face, the value of descorticoids, once recommended, has not been confirmed. In the case of meningeal involvement with no germ on direct examination, the combination of a 3rd-generation cephalosporin with fosfomycin and metronidazole is reasonable(20).

12.2   Symptomatic treatment:

2.1. **Anti-coma treatment** : reserved for forms with epileptic seizures. There is no preference for a particular molecule. The question of the duration of treatment remains unresolved. In our experience, treatment is usually continued for 1 year, then tapered off progressively in the absence of new seizures, and the electroencephalogram is normal.

2.2. **Treatment of intracranial hypertension** is usually medical. Corticosteroids have long been used, but acetazolamide and fluid restriction are now preferred. In cases of isolated ICH, lumbar puncture prior to heparin treatment, combined with acetazolamide, usually results in rapid improvement of headache and adequate control of visual function.

2.3. Finally, **analgesic treatment** is often indispensable in the acute phase, due to the sometimes intense headaches. These are usually rapidly improved by anticoagulant treatment, and major analgesics are generally unnecessary.

12.3 Anti-thrombotic treatment:

It is based on **heparin in anticoagulant dosage**. Long debated, the benefits of heparin are now accepted, even in cases of hemorrhagic lesions.

The first article on the subject was by Marie Germanwho found that, in a series of 38 patients, the 23 who received curative anticoagulant treatment all survived.

-A meta-analysis of anticoagulation studies has shown a benefit of anticoagulant treatment on the patient's vital and functional prognosis, albeit modest.

-In practice, anticoagulant therapy should be offered to all patients with definite CVT, including those with hemorrhagic infarction, as long as there are no contraindications to such treatment. The optimal duration of anticoagulant treatment is not precisely known (three to six months).

In practice, therefore, it is prescribed as soon as the diagnosis is confirmed. There is no consensus on the modalities, type (unfractionated heparin or low-molecular-weight heparin) or duration of heparin therapy.

After a few days, in the absence of clinical worsening, per os anticoagulants are generally administered, the duration of which depends on the underlying cause.

The use of **fibrinolytics** was proposed as early as 1971. No randomized studies are available. A recent meta-analysis analyzed data from 72 studies involving 169 patients. It highlighted the disparity in management: type of fibrinolytic used, route of administration (systemic or local), dosage, possible association with mechanical maneuvers.

The results showed a relatively good prognosis for thrombolysis patients, with a death or dependency rate of 12%, despite the fact that these were mostly severe forms of thrombolysis (coma: 32%; encephalopathy: 48%). Of course, these results must be interpreted with caution, due to probable publication bias and the absence of randomized studies.

Thrombolysis, with or without mechanical deobstruction maneuvers, is still the exception rather than the rule, and should be reserved for forms that worsen despite well-managed medical treatment, which in our experience accounts for around 5% of cases (14.15.20).

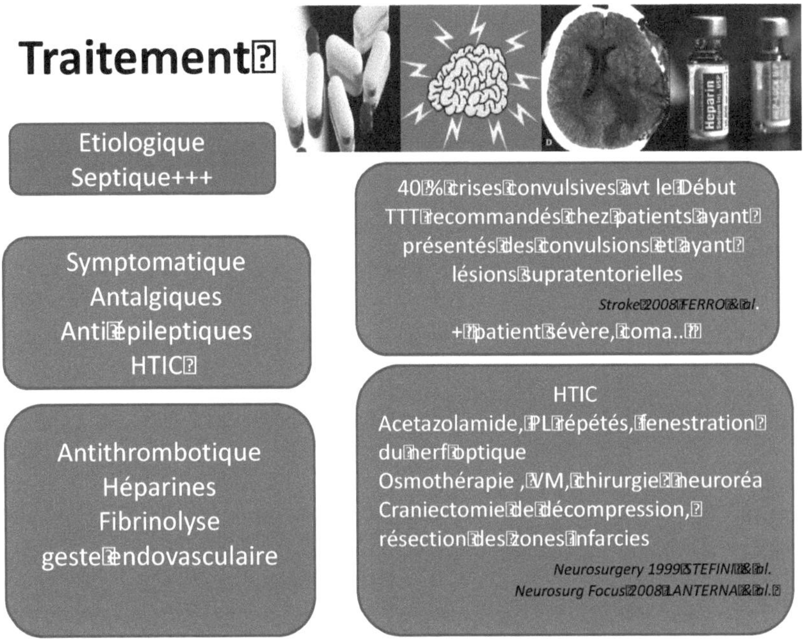

Figure 22: Main lines of treatment for DVTs

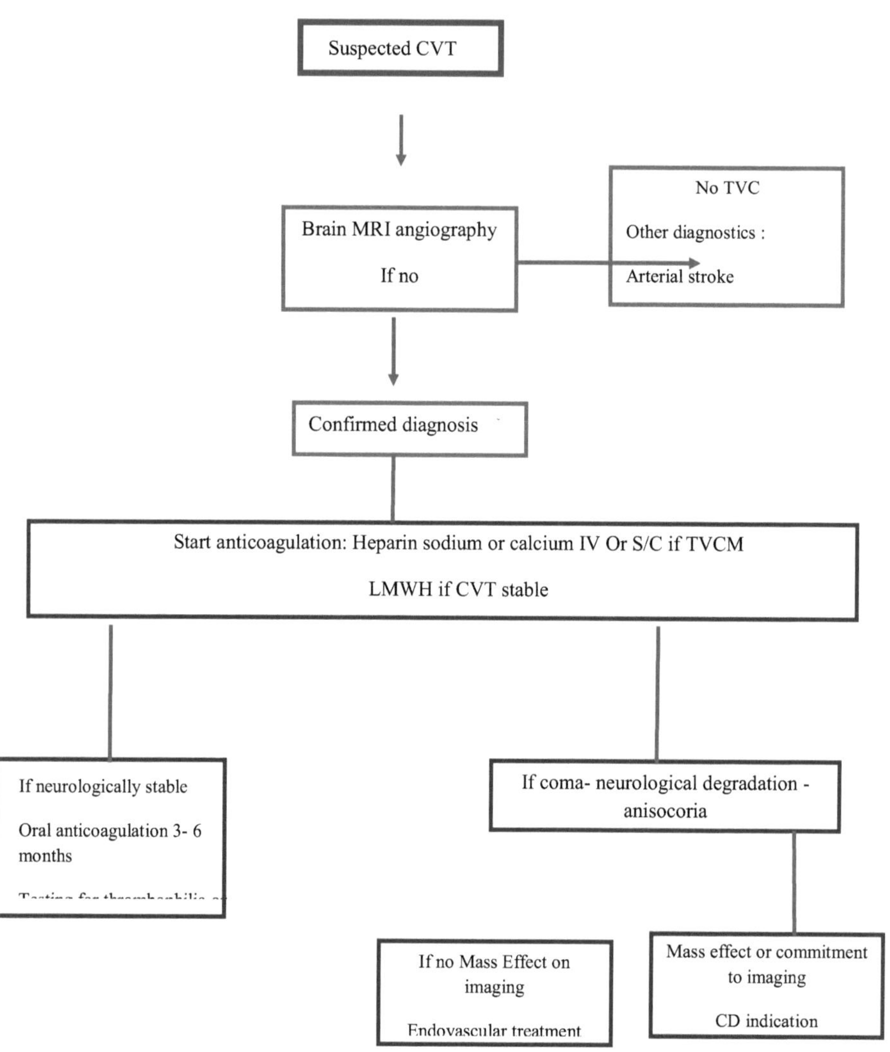

Figure 23: Global algorithm for the management of Cerebral Venous Thrombosis proposed by **Gustavo Saposnik et al. Stroke. 2011;42:1158-1192**

CVT: cerebral venous thrombosis - CMVT: malignant cerebral venous thrombosis - DC: decompressive craniotomy - LMWH: low molecular weight heparin

Clinical signs of CVT can range from simple headaches to focal neurological deficits and/or convulsions.

The literature reports that an uncommon and rapid presentation was found in ¼ of cases. This is a progressive malignant form where the patient rapidly deteriorates his neurological score and ends up in deep coma with or without pupillary dilatation.

This situation is explained by a combination of edema due to venous damage and intracerebral hemorrhage, leading to an increase in ICP.

Death in these patients is due to intracranial hypertension, so performing CD is sensible [30].

The first series of decompression surgery were described in the 1980s by Nagpal and colleagues. In a series of 70 TVCMs, 32 patients underwent this procedure. Survival was 54%, and improvement was observed in 89% of surgical survivors; death was due to delayed surgery [31].

Another study by Marie Théaudin involved 12 TVCMs who were comatose with pupillary changes and scannographic signs of involvement.

Eight patients had undergone surgical decompression: external in 4, external and internal in 3, and internal in only one.

The 4 patients who did not undergo surgery died within 1 to 5 days of diagnosis. One patient in the operated group died of a pulmonary embolism. The other 7 survived. The author of this article concludes that decompressive surgery can save lives and may even allow a good functional outcome in TVCM even in patients with bilateral dilated pupils. [32]

Gustavo Saposnik et al. in an article published in Stroke in 2011, proposed an algorithm for the management of CVT. In the event of suspected CVT, they recommend MRI. If the MRI is positive, treatment with heparin sodium or LMWH should be initiated. For neurologically stable patients, oral anticoagulants should be continued for 3 to 6 months, while the most severe patients should receive either endo-vascular treatment or CD. This management is illustrated in figure 23[33].

14 EVOLUTION AND PROGNOSIS :

Thanks to improved diagnostic possibilities and early treatment, the prognosis of CVT has improved markedly in recent years. Stroke patients usually recover without sequelae, with an acute mortality rate of 4.3%.

The predictive factors for death identified by multivariate analysis are :
- Coma on admission (Glasgow score<9
- Confusion;

- Epileptic seizures;

Before the introduction of angiography, the diagnosis of CVT was often an anatomical finding, which led to an overestimation of mortality. Today, the vast majority of CVTs have a favorable course, which explains their low incidence in autopsy series. Fatal cases have become rare, and death is more often related to the causative condition or pulmonary embolism than to the thrombosis itself(2). The following factors have a poor prognosis:

- age, with high mortality at the extremes of life (children and the elderly)
- the presence of focal signs or coma;
- existence of hemorrhagic infarction and delta sign on CT scan
- involvement of the deep venous system or posterior fossa veins
- recovery capacity is generally much greater than in arterial thrombosis. Sequelae occur in a small proportion of patients (around 20%) and consist mainly of focal deficits. There are also visual sequelae with post-stasis optic atrophy, which earlydiagnosis and treatment should be able to prevent. The long-term evolution is poorly understood.

14 CONCLUSION

Clinical diagnosis of CVT is difficult, due to the polymorphism of symptoms and course. It must often be made in an emergency situation, and requires neuroradiological examinations, ideally MRI/MVR.

Once treatment has been initiated, the disease is usually cured. Treatment is currently based on heparin, combined with etiological and symptomatic therapies tailored to each clinical situation.

However, it is important to be aware of the existence of severe forms, as certain prognostic factors can help identify them. Clinicians must keep in mind the possibility of excellent clinical recovery, and may propose more aggressive treatments such as in situ thrombolysis or mechanical clot-busting. However, their indications remain to be defined in a randomized trial.

The Messages in this book:

1. Unusual headache in a woman should prompt a diagnosis of CVT

2. Despite being widely documented in the literature, TVCs often go unrecognized.

3. Early diagnosis where headache, deficit and seizures are the most frequent signs

4. Clinical polymorphism

5. Beware of psychiatric forms that can lead to misdiagnosis

6. Angioscanner or injected CT scan should be performed in any patient presenting with neurological symptoms.

7. Angio-MRI is the most specific radiological examination for diagnosing this pathology.

8. Early anticoagulation improves prognosis

9. Anticoagulation even in the case of hemorrhagic lesions

10. Etiological treatment: antibiotics for sinusitis, mastoiditis and meningitis

11. Identify the most serious patients for whom decompression surgery should be discussed with the neurosurgeon

12. Pathology with an excellent prognosis if diagnosed early

BIBLIOGRAPHICAL REFERENCES S

1.   P. Reiner - I. Crassard - A.-C. Lukaszewicz. Cerebral venous thrombosis Réanimation (2013) 22:624-633 (2)

2.   José Manuel Ferro, PatríciaCanhão, Diana Aguiar de Sousa .Cerebralvenousthrombosis Presse Med. 2016; 45: e429-e450

3.   Thrombose veineuse cérébral .Feuillet de radiologie2006,46,n° 2 ,155-16 Masson paris 2006 Département d'Imagerie Morphologique et Fonctionnelle, Centre Hospitalie .Sainte- Anne,1, rue Cabanis, 7567 Paris Cedex.

4.   Vein thrombosis and cerebral sinusesLienerta, Hans-Werner Ottb a Abteilung Neurologie, MedizinischeUniversitätsklinik, Bruderholzspital, Bruderholb Institut für Radiologie, Bruderholzspital, Bruderholz CURRICULUM.

5.   ThromboseveineusecérébraleGuide   pratique   des   urgences neurovasculairesBousser MG, Mas JL (2009) Traité de neurologie. Accident vasculaire cérébraux. Éditions Doin 593-613.

6.   Cerebral   venous   thrombosiscrassardaameridrougemontmgBousser Encyclopédie Médico-Chirurgicale 17-046-R-10I

7.   Elalamy I. Mechanisms and risk factors of venous thrombosis. Encyclopédie médi-chirurgical(Editions Scientifiques et Médicales Elsevier SAS, Paris, all rights reserved 19-2095, 2002, 8 p Angiology Resident's Manual

8.   http://www.flashcardmachine.com/neuroanatomie.html

9.   Changing pattern of headache pointing to cerebral venous thrombosis after lumba puncture and intravenous high-dose corticosteroids.*Headache* 1999; 39: 559-64. PaidiS, Chaunu MP, Biousse V, Bousser.

10.   Feuillet de radiologie2006, 46, n° 2 ,155-1 Masson paris 2.

11.   Martinelli I. Risk factors in venous thromboembolism ThrombHaemost2001; 86: 395-403Bauer KA.Thethrombophilias well-defined risk factors with uncertain therapeutic implications.Anninternnmed2001; 135: 367-373Encyclopédie Médico-Chirurgicale 19-2095

12.   Cerebral venous thrombosis Martinelli I. Risk factors in venousthromboembolismThrombHaemost 2001; 86: 395-40 Manuel du resident angéologie.

13.   Venous   sinuses
http://www.chups.jussieu.fr/polys/neuranat/TDP2/POLY.Chp.1.3.html   Centre Hospitalier Universitaire de la Pitié Salpêtrière.
14.   Cerebral thrombophlebitis E. Maury, D. Lacroix, J. Chiras, G. OffenstReanimation

15.   Laurent Brunereau, Claude Lévy, Manuela Vasile, KathlynMarsot-Dupuch, Jean- Michel Tubiana, Radiology Department, Hôpital Saint-Antoinethrombose veinneuse cérébrale Author(s) :, 184, rue

16.   Du Faubourg- Saint-Antoine, 75012 Paris.

17.   Crahronbossard.Cerebral thrombophlebitis I Encyclopédie Médico-Chirurgicale 17-046-R-1

18.   Cerebral venous thrombosisR.AHDEB H.HOSSEI 2009 ALSEVIER MASSON SAS

19.   Cerebral venous thrombosis. Réanimation 2001 ; 10 : 383- © 2001 Éditions scientifiques et médicales Elsevier SAS. S11646756010013111/SSU

20.   RADIOLOGICAL IMAGING OF CEREBRAL THROMBOPHLEBITES Hôpitalpitj. CHIRASpitié-Salpétrière - Paris

21.   Diagnostic and therapeutic management of cerebral thrombophlebitis MATTEIS OLIVIER DESC Reanimation médicale de GRENOBLE 06/2006

22.   Cerebral venous thrombosis W. Meissner, I. Sibon, J.-M. Orgogozo, F Rouane

23.   Thrombosis of cerebral veins and sinuses Carmen Lienerta, Hans-Werner Ottb a Abteilung Neurologie, MedizinischeUniversitätsklinik, Bruderholzspital, Bruderholzzb Institut für Radiologie, Bruderholzspital, Bruderholz

24.   Cerebral venous thrombosis in the SAU Dr Perrine Ravasse, Dr Sandra Abergel, Dr Jean-Christophe Allo (SAU Cochin) Urgence online

25.   Cerebral venous thrombosisthe essential scientific and medical information John libbeyeurotext
26.   Management of cerebral venous thrombosisfrance Woimant USINV Lariboisière Paris
27.   Magnetic resonance angiography of cerebral venous thrombosis

28.   <u>Blood Thrombosis Vessels. Volume 7, Number 6, 385-94, June - July 1995, Mini-reviews</u>

29.   International Study on Cerebral Vein and Dural Sinus Thrombosis' 1998 -2001

30.   Ferro JM, Canhao P, Stam J, Bousser MG, BarinagarrementeriaF; ISCVT Investigators. Prognosis of cerebral vein and dural sinus thrombosis:results of the International Study on CerebralVein and Dural Sinus Thrombosis(ISCVT). Stroke. 2004;35:664-70.

31.   Nagpal RD. Dural sinus and cerebralvenousthrombosis. NeurosurgRev. 1983;6:155-60 [8] Théaudin M1, Crassard I, Bresson D, Saliou G, Favrole P, Vahedi K, Denier C, BousserMG.Shoulddecompressive surgery be performed in malignant cerebral venous thrombosis: a series of 12 patients. Stroke. 2010 Apr;41(4):727-31. doi10.1161/STROKEAHA.109.572909. Epub 2010 Feb 25.

32.   Saposnik G, Barinagarrementeria F, Brown RD Jr, et al; and the American Heart Association Stroke Council and the Council on Epidemiology and Prevention. (2011). Diagnosisand management of cerebralvenousthrombosis: a statement for healthcare

Cerebral Venous Thrombosis — A Review of 38 Cases

Marie-Germaine Bousser, M.D.,* Jacques Chiras, M.D.,†

Jacques Bories, M.D.,† and Paul Castaigne, M.D.*

SUMMARY A series of 38 patients with angiographically proven cerebral venous thrombosis (CVT) affecting dural sinuses is reported. This study shows that CVT is not rare, that the clinical diagnosis is extremely difficult because of the variable modes of onset and groupings of symptoms, that most CT findings are non specific and that angiography remains the best diagnostic tool. Only 4 patients died, which suggests a more benign outcome than classically described. None of the 23 heparin treated patients died, which indicates that anticoagulants were not harmful in this series.

Stroke Vol 16, No 2, 1985

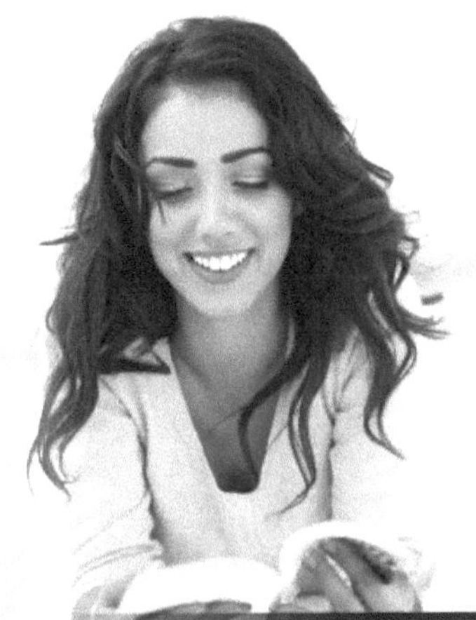

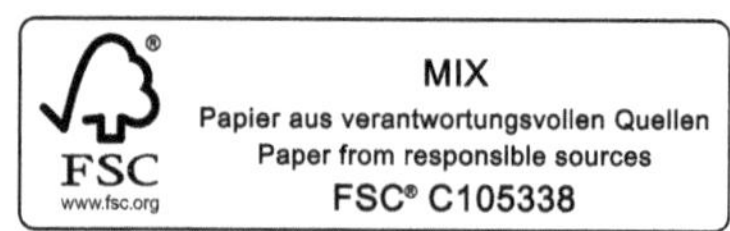

Printed by Books on Demand GmbH, Norderstedt / Germany